TEEN DRINKING

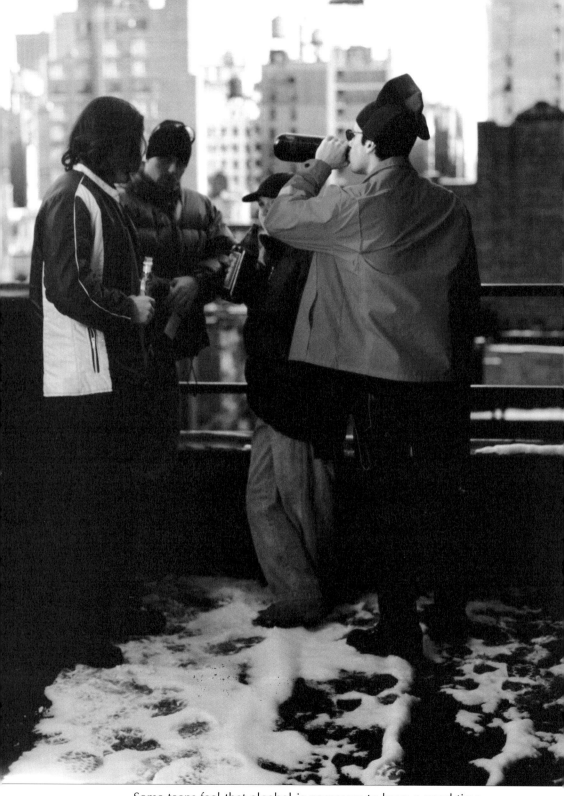

Some teens feel that alcohol is necessary to have a good time.

TEEN DRINKING

Christine Bichler

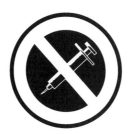

THE ROSEN PUBLISHING GROUP, INC.
NEW YORK

Published in 2000 by The Rosen Publishing Group, Inc.
29 East 21st Street, New York, NY 10010

First Edition

Library of Congress Cataloging-in-Publication Data

Bichler, Christine
  Teen drinking / by Christine Bichler.
    p.   cm.—(The drug abuse prevention library)
  Includes bibliographical references and index.
  Summary: Examines the issue of alcohol use among teens, including the physical and psychological effects of alcohol abuse, risk factors for alcoholism, and sources of help for teens at risk.
    ISBN 0-8239-2830-6
    1. Teenagers—Alcohol use—United States Juvenile literature. 2. Alcoholism—United States—Prevention Juvenile literature. 3. Alcohol—Physiological effect Juvenile literature. [1. Alcoholism.] I. Title. II. Series.
  HV5135.849 1999
    362.292'0835'0973—dc21   99-16886
                                                                CIP

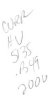

Contents

Introduction   *6*

Chapter 1   Alcohol Use   *11*

Chapter 2   Dangers of Alcohol Use   *22*

Chapter 3   Alcoholism   *33*

Chapter 4   Why Do People Drink?   *41*

Chapter 5   Choices to Make   *52*

Glossary   *58*

Where to Go for Help   *60*

For Further Reading   *62*

Index   *63*

Introduction

*F*ew people reach their teenage years in the United States without becoming aware of alcohol. It seems to be advertised everywhere—in magazines, on television. Rock and rap concerts are often sponsored by manufacturers of alcoholic beverages. Television commercials for beer make drinking seem like an essential part of hanging out with friends and having a good time. Movies and TV programs show successful people sipping wine or cocktails in fancy restaurants or average folks drinking beer with pals at the local bar where "everybody knows your name." You may see your parents and their friends relaxing with a beer, a glass of wine, or a

drink before dinner.

Alcohol has been part of human society for thousands of years. In many cultures, alcohol is used on important social occasions and in religious ceremonies. It is used to celebrate and to mourn, to seal friendships and business deals, and to lessen the pain of loneliness. In the United States, alcohol consumption seems to be such an ordinary part of everyday life that most people do not give much thought to it—and most people end up making the decision about whether to drink without really weighing all the positives and negatives.

Yet few decisions have such potentially serious consequences. Alcohol use is so common that it is easy to forget that alcohol is a drug—a very dangerous drug. For teens, it is also an illegal drug, which is also easy to forget. At present, every state and the District of Columbia prohibits the sale of alcohol to persons under the age of twenty-one. Though adults may use alcohol legally, alcohol use is still one of the most serious problems faced by our society. In the United States, alcohol is the most commonly used drug—and the most commonly abused. Each year, alcohol use contributes heavily to traffic fatalities, domestic violence, and the spread of the disease known as alcoholism,

8 which already affects millions of Americans. Alcohol use is often a factor in criminal behavior and in unplanned or unwanted sexual activity.

For teens especially, alcohol use affects decision making, which can result in poor choices that influence everything from physical and mental health to relationships with friends, family, and peers, as well as work and study habits and other issues that affect your future.

Young people are naturally curious about alcohol. Alcohol use has been a badge of adulthood in this country for generations. You may have heard your father talk about "keg parties" from his high school or college days. You may have been served wine or champagne at a cousin's wedding and noticed the tingly feeling that it gave you after you drank it. Maybe you have seen older brothers or sisters or cousins use alcohol. Many parents who would be horrified to find their children smoking pot or taking other drugs choose to ignore the fact that teenagers are drinking alcohol—perhaps because it is the drug they are most likely to use themselves.

This book is intended to inform you of the potential risks involved with drinking alcohol, so you can make informed decisions. It will discuss the ways that alcohol affects the body, talk about some of the reasons that people drink, and examine the health and safety issues most often associated with alcohol use. Whatever messages you receive from your friends, family, and the media, the decision of when and whether to start drinking is not a simple one. It is, however, one that only you can make. Be sure that you have all the facts before you make it.

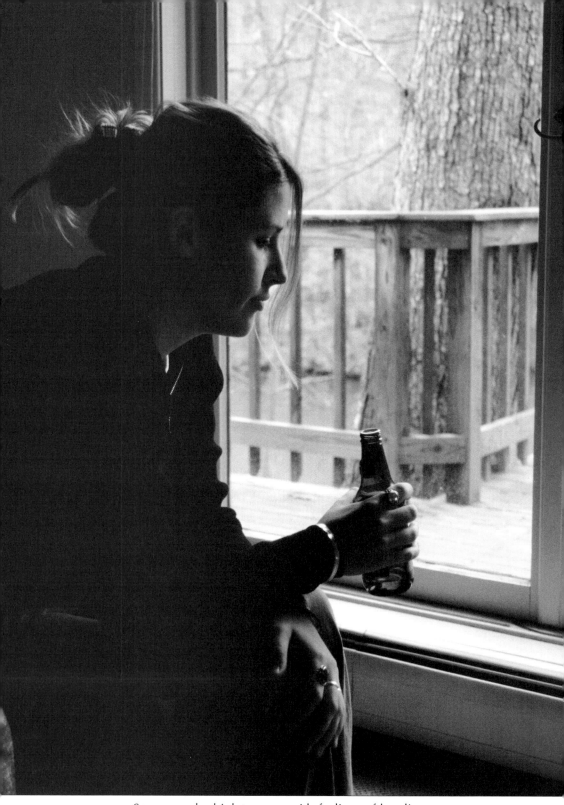

Some people drink to cope with feelings of loneliness.

CHAPTER 1

Alcohol Use

Kate arrived at the party feeling awkward and shy. As the new girl in her high school, she was surprised that she had even been invited. Although she had plenty of friends at her old school, she had never considered herself one of the popular crowd.

Kate looked around nervously. The room was filled with teenagers, laughing and chatting in small groups. A girl that Kate thought she recognized waved her over. "Don't I know you from art class?" the girl asked.

Kate smiled. "That's right—I'm Kate."

"I'm Julie," said the other girl. "I love what I've seen of your drawings. I meant to tell you that the other day. I'm glad to see you here."

Kate was relieved that she had someone to talk to who seemed to share her interests.

12   *Julie took Kate back to the kitchen, where a variety of snacks and drinks were spread out on the table. Julie went to the freezer and took out a pitcher of what looked like frozen punch. It was actually a margarita mix. "Since it's a special occasion, I made this. Want some?"*

Kate was not sure. She had never tried alcohol before. But this party seemed different from the "keggers" and wild parties she had heard about. Julie seemed very intelligent and mature. The idea of drinking alcohol did not seem to bother her, even though she was probably not much older than Kate, who was sixteen.

"There's plenty of other stuff here that's not alcoholic," said Julie. "I just thought you might want to try it. It tastes really good."

"I guess a little taste won't hurt me," agreed Kate. She took a swallow. The drink tasted like fruit, except it was bitter. It fizzed like soda pop and caused a slight burning sensation on its way to her stomach.

Kate spent the rest of the evening talking to Julie and meeting her friends. She finished her first margarita and began a second one. In a few hours, she found herself talking easily with everyone in the room, even flirting a little with the good-looking boys at the party. She had never been brave enough to do that before. She wondered if alcohol was making

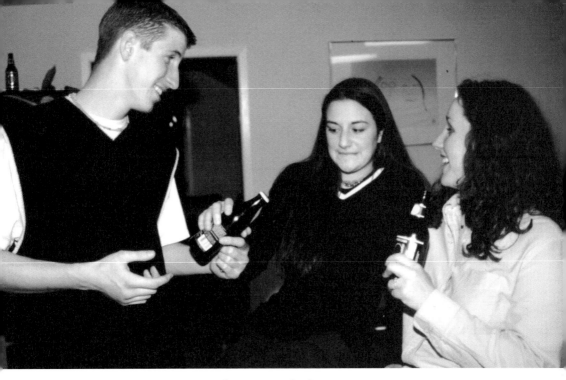

Sometimes it can seem as if everyone drinks.

her bolder. For a minute, she even wondered if she might be drunk, or on her way to getting drunk. But Kate did not feel out of control, just a little more outgoing than usual—a bit lightheaded, maybe, but not in a bad way. "Maybe I just needed a drink to relax me," Kate thought.

Many people, both adults and teenagers, have had experiences like Kate's—using alcohol to loosen up and relax at a party. Obviously, many people find using alcohol pleasurable in some ways, or else its use would not be so common. What is equally obvious is that both short- and long-term use of alcohol can have many negative consequences. The best way to understand

13

14 | these effects is to examine the way alcohol affects the body.

What Is Alcohol?

Alcohol is the common name for a substance known as ethyl alcohol, which is created through a process called fermentation. In fermentation, grain, fruit, honey, or other foods containing sugar are mixed with yeast. The yeast, which is a living organism, consumes the sugar and produces carbon dioxide along with ethyl alcohol. Beer, wine, wine coolers, and so-called "hard" or distilled liquors, such as whiskey, rum, and vodka, all contain alcohol.

Alcohol is a drug. Drugs are chemicals that people put into their bodies in order to bring about some change in their mental or physical state. Not all drugs are illegal. The majority of drugs have some medicinal purpose. Aspirin, for example, is the trade name for a manufactured version of a drug—acetylsalicylic acid—that relieves pain. You may have taken aspirin to relieve a headache or other cold symptoms, or to relieve pain from an injury.

Drugs that have medical uses can be bought in a pharmacy or drugstore, either over-the-counter, such as aspirin, or with

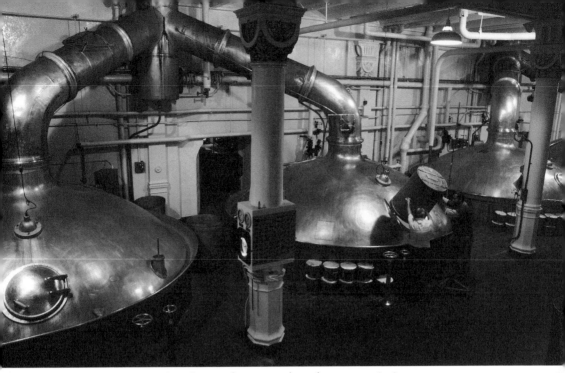

Fermentation is the chemical process that changes grain into ethyl alcohol.

a prescription from a doctor. Most drugs that have little or no legitimate medical use, such as heroin and cocaine, are illegal. This means that their sale, possession, or use can result in arrest and a jail sentence or other legal penalty. Unlike these substances, the use of alcohol is legal for people older than twenty-one in the United States. But like heroin and cocaine, alcohol is dangerous and addictive.

Like these illegal drugs, alcohol is a psychoactive drug—a drug that alters the way you think and feel. Unlike heroin and cocaine, alcoholic beverages can provide minimal value to the body through calories, but generally they are consumed for the pleasurable sensation or "high" they give

16 | the user. When alcoholic beverages are consumed, even in small amounts, they often produce an increased sense of well-being and sociability. Some studies have even indicated that moderate use of alcohol—no more than the equivalent of one or two glasses of wine a day with dinner—may have some positive health effects for certain people. There is no doubt, however, that larger amounts of alcohol can be damaging and even deadly.

The Effects of Alcohol

Alcohol is not digested like food. Instead, it is absorbed directly into the bloodstream through the stomach and small intestine. From there, it moves to the brain and other parts of the body. For most people, it does not take long to feel the effects of drinking even a small amount of alcohol.

In small amounts, alcohol acts as a stimulant. It makes people feel more lively, cheerful, and active by seeming to speed up certain body functions. Many people feel more talkative or outgoing after a couple of drinks, less shy, wittier, and more charming. They may even feel they are thinking more clearly. Other people also often appear more attractive to the drinker.

In reality, however, alcohol functions as

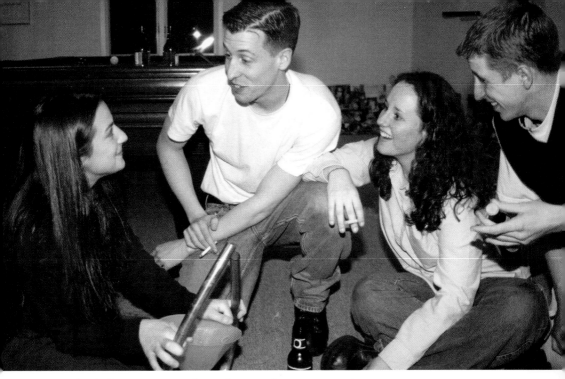

Alcohol use can initially make people more outgoing.

a depressant, or "downer," meaning that it slows down the brain and central nervous system. In the process, alcohol lessens an individual's control of his body, thoughts, and emotions. The "pick-up" or stimulant effect that some people enjoy from alcohol is in fact a loosening of inhibitions and self-control as a result of alcohol's strength as a depressant. Reflexes, reactions, and responses—both the physical and mental kind—become slowed and less reliable.

One result: You feel less shy or self-conscious in company after a couple of beers. Another: You feel embarrassed or humiliated the next day about something you have said or done while using alcohol—something you would never have

18 | said or done if you had not been drinking. Some degree of memory loss is a common side effect of alcohol use. Such loss extends all the way to blackouts—total loss of memory about one's actions while under the influence of alcohol—which can result from excessive alcohol use.

As more alcohol is consumed, an individual becomes drunk, or intoxicated, as alcohol causes the brain to lose more and more control over the body. People who have had too much to drink often exhibit symptoms such as slurred speech, loss of muscle control, and delayed reactions to what is going on around them. Some become morose or withdrawn, overly emotional, sad, or weepy. Others proceed from jovial or boisterous behavior to aggressive or belligerent "acting out." Sometimes excessive drinking causes people to lose consciousness.

Alicia was not sure how many beers she had drunk. But after a while, the sensations became unmistakable—she was going to throw up. She stumbled to the bathroom just in time to vomit into the toilet. Meanwhile, the party continued outside. The loud music made her head throb. Other people were laughing, and she wondered if they were laughing at her. "Great," she thought, "That's the way to get

yourself noticed. Act like a drunk." She felt
awful. The room seemed to be tilting. Her body was shaking. There was nothing to do but hug the toilet and hope the sensations would pass. How was she ever going to explain this to her parents? She knew they would be able to tell she had been drinking. She would be in trouble, grounded forever. "How did this happen to me?" she wondered. "It was only a few beers."

It is not uncommon for drinkers, especially new drinkers who are not used to the effects of alcohol, to get sick from ingesting it. Vomiting is one way that your body gets rid of harmful substances.

And if you are not sick right away, you may be later. One of the most unpleasant aspects of alcohol use is the hangover experienced by drinkers on the dreaded "morning after." Hangover symptoms include headache, fever, chills, muscle ache, nausea, fatigue, insomnia, and depression. Hangovers generally become worse as one recalls—or is reminded of—one's unwise behavior from the night before.

Alcohol Use in the United States Today

You may have heard politicians speak about the "war on drugs," or heard counselors

20 talk about the subject, or seen advertisements or stories about it in the media. What you are less likely to have heard is that America's greatest drug problem is with alcohol.

Because alcohol use is so commonplace, its devastating effects are easy to overlook. That it is so common only makes teenagers' decisions about drinking that much more complicated. By the time you start thinking about whether—and how—you are going to use alcohol, you may have already been profoundly affected by alcohol's misuse. And you would not be alone. It is estimated that 76 million Americans, or nearly half (43 percent) of the adult U.S. population, have been exposed to alcoholism in their own families.

This is not surprising when you consider that one out of every eight Americans who uses alcohol suffers from the chronic, severe, and devastating fatal disease known as alcoholism. The financial cost to American society of such alcohol abuse is immense—an estimated $170 billion each year.

There is a hidden cost that is even greater. Twenty-eight million Americans—one out of every eight—are children of alcoholics (COAs). More than ten million COAs are young men and women under the age of eighteen. These individuals are at great risk of experiencing the most severe dangers of alcohol and other drug use. No one is immune, however, and there is no excuse for not being informed.

CHAPTER 2

Dangers of Alcohol Use

*K*ate noticed a group of kids clustered together at the other end of the room. They were a little older, were talking loudly, laughing a lot—and drinking a lot. Kate took Julie aside. "I don't think I've ever met those people before."

"Oh—they're seniors—Mark and those guys. They're looking forward to graduating. That guy over there, Brad Summers—he just got accepted into the University of Michigan."

"Why so much booze?" asked Kate. "Doesn't that make you a little nervous?"

"Oh, Mark's always getting toasted—but don't worry. He'll pass out soon—he's more pleasant when he's not making any noise."

Julie was right. Fifteen minutes later, Mark passed out on the floor amid a pile of beer cans. The other kids didn't even seem to notice.

After a while, Kate heard someone say, *"Geez, he's really wasted—he doesn't even look like he's breathing." Someone else took a look. "Wait a minute," a young man said. "I really don't think he is."*

"Yeah, right."

"I'm serious—I don't think he's breathing."

Panic spread. "We can't call 911—my parents will freak."

"The cops . . . "

Standing in a corner, Kate had never been so terrified. Finally, Julie called an ambulance.

Binge Drinking

An extreme example? Maybe. But it does happen, maybe more often than you think. When most people think of sudden death resulting from alcohol use, they think of automobile accidents. Such incidents certainly are among the most common and tragic associated with alcohol use. But as is true of any other drug, you can overdose on alcohol—fatally. What makes this possibility particularly frightening is that an estimated 2.6 million teenagers do not know that a person can die from an alcohol overdose. Julie had enough sense to call an ambulance. Would you?

General inexperience with alcohol use puts teens at a greater risk of overdosing.

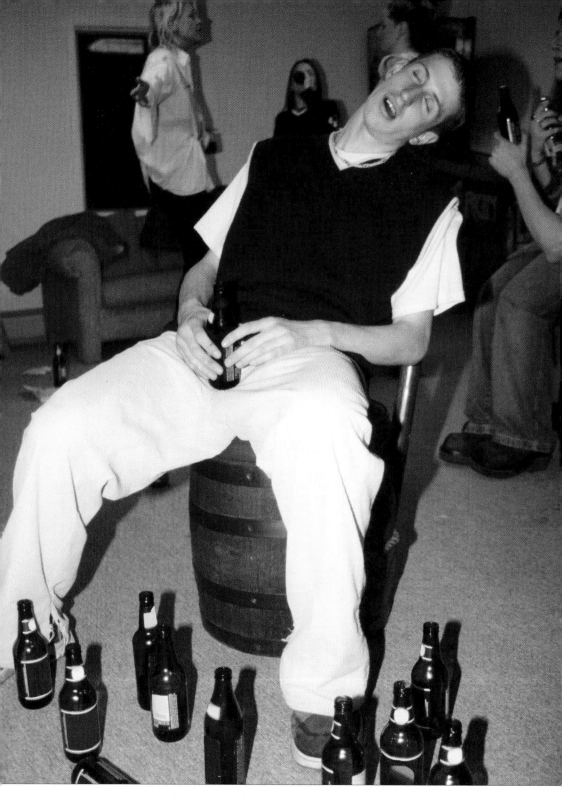

Binge drinking can lead to a potentially fatal alcohol overdose.

So does binge drinking, which is what Mark was doing. Binge drinking is especially popular among college students, but the practice has also spread to high schools. "Bingeing" refers to consuming lots of alcohol within a very short time period—five or more drinks in a row, often within just a couple of hours.

Excessive alcohol consumption puts a strain on your liver, which is the organ in your body that metabolizes, or burns up, the alcohol circulating in your bloodstream.

This process takes time, however. If you weigh 150 pounds, it can take your liver up to two hours to metabolize the alcohol from just one drink. If you continue to drink during those two hours, the metabolizing process takes even longer and makes your liver work even harder.

An overdose happens when the liver can no longer keep up with the amount of poison being poured into the body. The body simply shuts down, and death from heart or respiratory failure can be the result.

In other words, binge drinkers sometimes simply pass out and never wake up. Often, their friends do not bother to call for help because they do not realize that anything is wrong—they think that the intoxicated person just needs some time to "sleep off"

26 | the effect of the booze. In recent years, the number of such deaths has been rising.

Drunk Driving

Because alcohol interferes with awareness, judgment, vision, coordination, and reaction time, it impairs your ability to perform any complex activity, such as driving a car.

Driving while intoxicated or impaired—drunk driving—is dangerous, illegal, and a major public safety problem. The number of deaths from drunk driving has declined in recent years, but it remains the leading killer of teenagers in the United States.

Even a small amount of alcohol in the bloodstream affects your ability to drive. In most states, adults over twenty-one are considered to be driving while intoxicated or impaired (DWI) when they have .10 percent alcohol in their bloodstream. This is actually a fairly large amount, equal to two or three drinks for an average-sized adult man.

But driving with even a smaller amount of alcohol in your bloodstream—driving while under the influence of alcohol (DUI)—is illegal. Drinking and driving is a criminal offense, not just a traffic violation. Penalties vary from state to state, but they can be severe and include arrest and the suspension of your driver's license. |

Most important, however, is that if you drink and drive, you put yourself, passengers, and other drivers at risk of serious injury or death. In the United States, eight young people die each day in alcohol-related crashes. More than 40 percent of all deaths from automobile accidents involve alcohol. More than 40 percent of the deaths of sixteen- to twenty-year-olds result from car crashes, and alcohol use is involved in more than half of those fatal accidents. In fact, when a sixteen-year-old dies in the United States, the death is probably related in some way to alcohol use.

Remember that you do not have to get into a car with someone who has been drinking. If you know that your friends will be drinking at a gathering, you can volunteer to be the "designated driver," stay alcohol-free, and drive everyone home safely. If your friends insist on drinking and driving, don't ride with them. Call a cab, your parents, or a friend. Better yet, avoid situations where drinking and driving is likely to occur.

Other Dangers

Of course, alcohol use is risky even if you do not drink and drive. What are some of the other dangers of alcohol use?

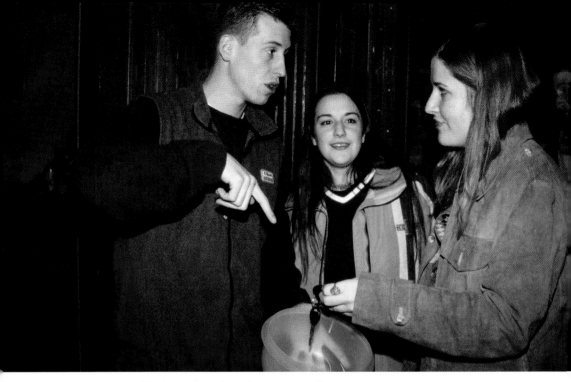

Designated, sober drivers save lives.

Simply put, alcohol threatens your life and health. There is the risk of sudden death or severe injury from overdose or automobile accidents. Alcohol use also puts you at much greater risk for other kinds of accidents. Alcohol use is involved in half of all boating accidents and more than half of all drownings. Nearly half of all deaths and serious injuries in the workplace involve alcohol use. Alcoholics are much more likely to die in falls or be the victims of accidental fires than other people.

Overall, alcohol contributes to 100,000 disease-related deaths each year in the United States, making it the third leading "preventable killer." And though cancer and heart disease kill more people each year, alcohol-related deaths occur at a much younger age. And alcohol is often a contributing factor to deaths from heart disease and cancer.

Too dramatic? Consider alcohol's long-term health consequences. Alcohol use harms virtually every organ and system in the human body. It is the major cause of diseases of the liver and pancreas. It contributes greatly to high blood pressure and stroke. In both women and men, it causes various serious problems with the reproductive system.

And if you do not want to think that far ahead, consider right now. You're in school for a reason, right? Well, nothing is more likely than alcohol to interfere with your education. Alcohol use is involved in 40 percent of all academic problems and 28 percent of all dropouts. If you are looking ahead to college and beyond, students with low averages (Ds and Fs) drink, in general, three times as much as students with As. Of all the students in college today in the United States, more will ultimately die of alcohol-related causes than will earn a graduate degree.

Finally, alcohol poses its greatest threat not to any specific system of your body but to something harder to define—your judgment. And ultimately, your judgment is all

30 you have to rely on to strengthen and protect every area of your life. The same qualities of alcohol that help you act less shy also impair your ability to make decisions, which leads to bigger problems than just the memory of embarrassing behavior.

Yes, using alcohol at a party might make it easier to meet and talk with that cute guy or girl you find attractive. It also makes it harder to determine what kind of impression you are making on that person. It can also lead to more than talking, in the form of unwanted sexual activity, and to risky behavior concerning even desired sexual activity. For example, alcohol use is involved in up to two-thirds of all sexual assaults and date rape cases among teenagers and college students. A recent survey even showed that an alarming 39 percent of males (and 18 percent of females) believe that it is okay for a boy to force sex upon a girl if she is under the influence of alcohol or other drugs.

Even when sexual activity is consensual, alcohol use increases the risks involved. Among teenagers who are sexually active, those who are heavy drinkers are three times less likely to use condoms during sex. Such behavior greatly increases the risk of unwanted pregnancy or infection from the

HIV virus or other sexually transmitted diseases. Of all teens who drink, a significant portion of those who do regularly use condoms are less likely to do so after using alcohol. Among college women diagnosed with a sexually transmitted disease (STD), 60 percent were drunk at the time of infection.

Of course, forcing sex upon someone is a crime, regardless of whether that person is under the influence of alcohol. The poor decision-making that leads to criminal actions is made more likely by alcohol use. Also made more likely by the use of alcohol is the possibility that you will be the victim of a crime. Alcohol use by the offender and/or the victim is found in about half of all murders and criminal assaults and a high percentage of sex crimes, robberies, and domestic violence incidents. About 30 percent of the youths under age eighteen who are jailed for criminal acts are under the influence of alcohol at the time of arrest. Almost half of all college students who are victims of crime on campus are under the influence of alcohol or other drugs at the time of the incident. Alcohol use makes you more vulnerable to crime, because you are less aware of your surroundings when intoxicated and therefore an easier target for criminals.

32   Don't like to think of *yourself* as a criminal? Who does? But if you have ever driven a car while under the influence of alcohol, you already are one—by law.

There is one last thing to consider if you think alcohol is not as dangerous as other drugs because its use is common and legal. Alcohol is the substance most likely to act as a "gateway" drug. Teens who use alcohol are almost eight times as likely to use other drugs as teens who do not. Teens who drink are fifty times more likely to use cocaine. And like the users of any drug, those who use alcohol are susceptible to the downward spiral that leads from use to dependence to addiction.

CHAPTER 3

Alcoholism

Jamie is worried, though he hates to admit it. Like a lot of his friends, he has chosen to experiment with alcohol. But for Jamie, drinking seems to be different somehow. When he goes out with his friends, Jamie seems to drink more than they do. Or if he does not drink more, he definitely seems to get more drunk.

And he drinks more often than they do. When the group makes plans, it is usually Jamie who first suggests that they involve alcohol. Jamie has been making some new friends, but the only thing he really has in common with them is that they like to party as much as he does.

Sometimes, Jamie thinks that his old friends have started to treat him differently.

34 *They assume he is always going to get drunk when they are together, and they do not seem to take him as seriously. At parties he is treated like a clown, as if he gets intoxicated just to entertain others.*

Jamie does not drink all the time, so he knows he cannot be an alcoholic. Besides, he is too young for that, isn't he? But it seems like drinking and alcohol take up a lot more of his time, energy, and thoughts than they ever did before. He thinks about the last time he drank, and when he is going to drink again, and how come he seems to drink more—and more often—than other people.

"I'm not an alcoholic," he thinks, "so how can I have a problem with alcohol? I've never wrecked a car or been arrested, and my grades are good." Even so, all the questions and guilt and the confusion continue, even when he is drinking, which only seems to make him drink more. And then the questions get even harder to answer.

The Slippery Slope

Is Jamie an alcoholic? Without more information, it is hard to say. Does he have a problem with alcohol? Almost certainly. Is he too young to have such a problem? Certainly not. Jamie is somewhere on the slippery slope that leads downward from drug use to tolerance to dependency to addiction. With alcohol, that addiction is the disease known as alcoholism, and it is the number one drug problem among teenagers in the United States.

Chemical Dependency

Alcoholism is a form of chemical dependency. In this case, the chemical or drug upon which one becomes dependent is alcohol.

Most people go through similar stages on the way to chemical dependency. Most drug users have experiences that are similar, if not exactly the same. Chemical dependency is a process that varies by individual. With alcoholism, the process occurs something like this:

1. You begin experimenting with alcohol, for any number of possible reasons.
2. Your tolerance for alcohol increases. You need to drink more to achieve the same effect.
3. You experience memory lapses or blackouts. There are times when you do not remember what you did when you were drinking.
4. You avoid talking about alcohol. As your dependency increases, you try to divert attention away from it.

36

5. At the same time, you become preoccupied with alcohol. You spend an increasing amount of time thinking about drinking, plan your alcohol use carefully, and begin choosing your friends based on their alcohol use.
6. You make excuses for your alcohol use and even blame others for it. You use any reason as an excuse to drink. This stage is called denial.
7. You begin to lose control of your use of alcohol—when you drink, how much, how often, with whom.
8. Your alcohol use affects your relationship with your family or friends.
9. You start having new difficulties at school or your job. You may have medical or legal problems.
10. You begin to lose hope. As your addiction gets even worse, you start to feel that there is nothing that you can do about it.

The Two Types of Dependency

There are two types of chemical dependency—physical and psychological. Like some other drugs, alcohol causes both. Physical dependence is when a person's body needs alcohol in order for him or her to feel "normal"; the body reacts in a variety of ways to the lack of alcohol. The person may show physical symptoms of withdrawal when he or she cannot get alcohol. Such symptoms include shaking, sweating, irritability, confusion, and even hallucinations.

A person who is psychologically dependent on alcohol does not believe that he or she can live without it. The addict has a compulsive need to use alcohol. This need can occur either out of desire for alcohol's pleasurable effects or fear of withdrawal symptoms.

A Dangerous Disease

The form of chemical dependency or addiction known as alcoholism is a chronic and dangerous disease. Left untreated, its effects can be devastating, and they can lead to death.

It can be extremely difficult to tell whether someone is suffering from the disease of alcoholism. Most alcoholics are not homeless "winos" or "skid row" bums. Some people believe that in order to be an alcoholic, a person has to drink all or most of the time. This is not true.

Most alcoholics are like anyone else in your community—they have jobs and families, or they may go to school. It is possible

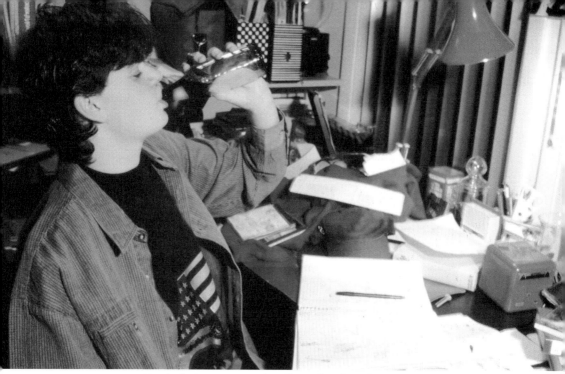
Alcohol abuse seriously affects family relationships.

to become an alcoholic at a very young age and very soon after beginning to experiment with alcohol. It is very possible for teenagers to develop a problem with alcohol use or even to become addicted. You may know someone with a drinking problem—a parent or even a classmate. You may even be concerned that you are developing an alcohol problem.

For an alcoholic, drinking gradually becomes the focus of his or her life. Alcoholics need to spend increasing amounts of time feeling the effects of alcohol, and they often need to consume increasing amounts of it to feel those effects. People who drink when they are upset, or to escape from their problems, or because

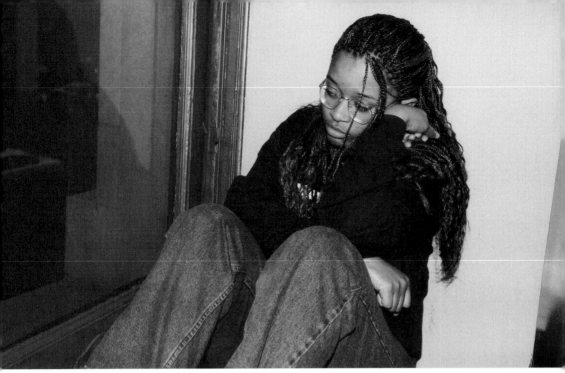

It is unwise—and dangerous—to turn to alcohol when you are unhappy.

they are unhappy, are at serious risk of becoming alcoholics.

Signs of Alcoholism

An important way to determine if a person is becoming an alcoholic is to see whether drinking is interfering with major areas of that person's life, such as school, health, family, or work. Has alcohol use taken the place of other activities or interests that once were important to that person? If you are starting to get into legal, financial, or academic trouble because of your drinking, if you cannot have fun without drinking, if you drink when you are upset or sad or troubled about something, if you drink as a

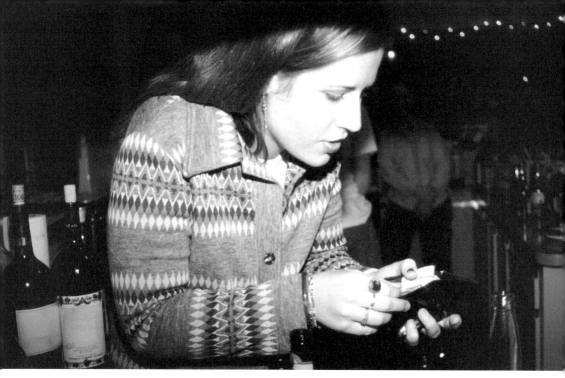

Financial problems caused by drinking can be an early sign of alcoholism.

way of "handling" your problems or as a way to avoid facing your problems, or if drinking has become an important "goal" in your life, you are in danger of becoming an alcoholic.

CHAPTER 4

Why Do People Drink?

Joseph has not felt right since his dad left. It feels as if there is a hole inside of him, and his stomach hurts all the time. He tries to concentrate at school, and that helps him forget his pain a little bit, but every afternoon, at the start of seventh period, he remembers that his father will not be there when he goes home, and he starts to feel bad again.

Joseph's mother said that they would be happier like this, and it is nice not to have to listen to his parents argue. But his mom seems even more unhappy now, and Joseph can tell that she worries a lot about money.

Joseph tries not to show that he is scared and sad about all of this. He is the oldest, after all, and he needs to show his little sisters and brother that things will be all right. His

42 | *mother has enough other stuff to worry about. Besides, lots of kids he knows do not have both of their parents living at home. Some of his schoolmates have hardly ever seen or known their dad. Bad things happen to everyone, right? he thinks. It doesn't do any good to talk about them.*

So Joseph never talks to his friends about what is happening at home, and he never talks about how he feels about it—except when he and his friends drink. Then he talks, and sometimes he even cries. His friends listen to him, and sometimes they tell him about things they have gone through. It feels good to talk to his friends like this, and he feels close to them, and he feels as though they can help each other. And so he does not feel quite so alone and sad all the time.

But he feels bad about the drinking, too. He wonders why he cannot seem to talk like this to anyone when he is not using alcohol. When his dad was drinking, that was when most of the fights started. Joseph worries, because he knows he himself is starting to drink more often than ever. He tells himself that this is going to change, but it is a funny thing: Ever since his dad left, the house seems smaller. Sometimes at night he feels like the walls of the house are closing in on him, and he just has to get out of there and

do something. And what he does is drink. It
seems to help, sort of.

Considering all that you have learned about the dangers of alcohol use, you might wonder why anyone would drink. There are probably as many specific reasons as there are people who drink. It would be nice to think that every alcohol user has made a careful, informed decision that the pleasures or benefits that he or she gets from alcohol outweigh any risks that come with its use. But what makes alcohol so dangerous, and its abuse so common, is that it interferes with your ability to make rational decisions about its use. And for many, many people, that process of destruction begins with the very first drink they ever take.

Why Teens Drink

Teenagers are in the process of trying out various adult roles and behaviors. The teen years are a period of learning about, experimenting with, and preparing for all kinds of adult activity. Alcohol use is one of these activities. Teens cannot help seeing the ways that adults use alcohol. Alcohol is used at times of great joy— such as a wedding celebration. It is also

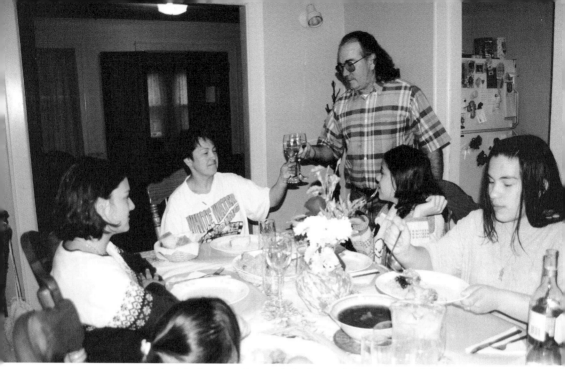

Alcohol is frequently used during celebrations and family gatherings.

used at times of great sadness—for example, when friends come together to mourn a death. It might be used as part of a social ritual that brings people together—family dinnertime at home, a meal at a restaurant with friends, a business lunch to seal a deal. It is used to stimulate social interaction—at clubs and bars where people go to dance, listen to music, and meet other people. It is used to relax after a long day at work, and to wash away many of the disappointments and realities of daily living.

So it is no surprise that many teens associate using alcohol with growing up and being considered an adult, and with the

challenge of adult responsibilities. Along | **45**
with dating, working, driving a car, and
voting, alcohol use can seem like a natural
part of growing up—and an eagerly antic-
ipated adult pleasure. In this sense, curios-
ity about alcohol and its effects is a natural
thing. With so much evidence of the large
role that alcohol use plays in adult society,
you may find yourself thinking, "Adults
drink—why shouldn't I?"

All in the Family

But teens use alcohol for many other
reasons than simply as a rite of passage
into adulthood. Anyone who uses alcohol,
for any reason, is at some risk of dependency, but some reasons that teens drink
make that danger much greater.

Problems within the family are the
most likely reason that teens turn to
alcohol. Such problems include physical,
emotional, or sexual abuse by a parent or
other family member. One or more
parents may be absent because of divorce,
death, or other reasons. Parents who are
not happy together can be an enormous
source of tension and stress for their children. Financial difficulties, emotional
strains, job demands, or their own drug or
alcohol use can cause even those parents

46 who are trying their best to become neglectful in different ways.

Such pressures within the family can lead to emotional problems for teens, such as depression or anxiety disorders. Lesser symptoms include intense feelings of loneliness, nervousness, and sadness. Often without realizing exactly what they are doing, many drug users, especially teens, use drugs and alcohol as a kind of self-medication for such problems.

Peer Pressure

Like everyone else, teens want to fit in. They want to have friends, to feel like they belong, to be considered smart and attractive by those their own age. This very natural desire also makes them susceptible to peer pressure.

A peer is a member of the same group to which you belong. In the broadest terms, all teenagers might be considered your peers. Or you might consider your peers to be those who go to the same school as you, or live in the same neighborhood, or are part of a particular group to which you belong or want to belong. Peer pressure is the pressure felt by members of that group, or by those who want to be considered members, to act or behave in a way that is accepted by the group.

For teens who are figuring out who they are by trying out many of the different kinds of adult behavior, peer pressure can be hard to resist. To go against peer pressure can mean being excluded from the group.

For teens with problems within their family, peer pressure can be even greater. Acceptance from peers may fill emotional needs that are not met at home or elsewhere. The support needed from within the family for the hard decisions that teens must make is often not available. Teens who are in situations that lead them to alcohol use often exert pressure on others to act the same way, sometimes without really intending to do so. Teens from similar backgrounds often become friends and behave in similar ways. Thus, it is easy for teens to feel that "everyone" they know drinks or uses drugs, and that to choose not to do so is to be left out.

Who Is at Risk?

No one intends to become an alcoholic or to have problems with the use of alcohol. And many people who use alcohol do so responsibly, without causing themselves or those they care about any great harm. But anyone who uses alcohol at all does risk problems. Clearly, there are some factors that put some people at a greater risk than others for developing problems with alcohol. How do you know if you are one of those at risk?

You are at risk if:

- You are young. First use of alcohol typically begins at age thirteen. A recent survey revealed that almost 70 percent of eighth graders and nearly 90 percent of twelfth graders have tried alcohol. Alcohol and other drug use at an early age is one of the best indicators of future drug or alcohol problems.
- You are uninformed. Eighty percent of teenagers do not know that there is as much alcohol in a can of beer or a glass of wine as there is in a shot of hard liquor.
- You use alcohol now. The only foolproof way that you can exercise control over the risks associated with alcohol use is not to drink, ever. Scientific evidence also shows that the younger you are when you begin using alcohol, the more likely it is that you will have problems related to its use. People who begin using alcohol before age

fifteen are four times more likely to become alcoholics than those who begin at twenty-one.

- A parent or close relative is an alcoholic or drug addict. Children of alcoholics are three to four times more likely to become alcoholics than children of non-alcoholics. Up to 25 percent of COAs are likely to become alcoholics. COAs are also much more likely to experience other forms of drug dependency. The reason for this may be both genetic and environmental. Some scientists believe that alcoholic parents can pass on a higher risk for the disease and other forms of chemical dependency to their children in their genes. And like any other behavior, alcohol use can be learned. A child who grows up in an environment where alcohol and drugs are misused is strongly influenced to behave in the same way.
- You are white. Whites are much more likely than African Americans, Hispanics, or members of other minority groups to use alcohol.
- You are male. Males are much more likely than females to use

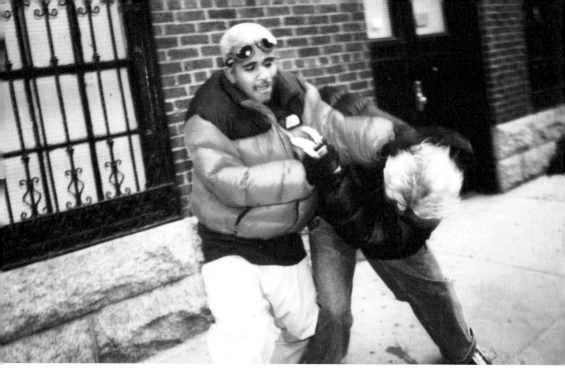

Alcohol use can lead to criminal or violent behavior.

alcohol and to become dependent
on it. White males drink far more
than any other group.

- You are female. Studies suggest that
women's bodies do not metabolize
alcohol as well as men's. Women also
tend to be physically smaller than
men. This leads to higher blood con-
centrations of alcohol over shorter
periods of time. This may also make
women more vulnerable to liver
disease caused by alcohol use.

- You use alcohol to cope with
shyness, family troubles, stress, or
other difficulties. Although it may
seem as if it helps, alcohol use is not

a way of addressing your problems.
Unaddressed problems do not go
away—they get worse. And if your
problems worsen, what is going to
happen to your alcohol use?

CHAPTER 5

Choices to Make

You have been given a lot of information. Information means knowledge, and knowledge leads to freedom and power—power to control your decisions about alcohol use, instead of letting alcohol use control your decisions.

What Should You Do?
That is up to you. But if you are using alcohol, and you think that you may have a problem with it, then you do. If any aspect of your alcohol use is troubling you at all, you should strongly consider getting help or advice. There is no such thing as being too young to have a problem with alcoholism or any other form of chemical dependency. You shouldn't wait until you

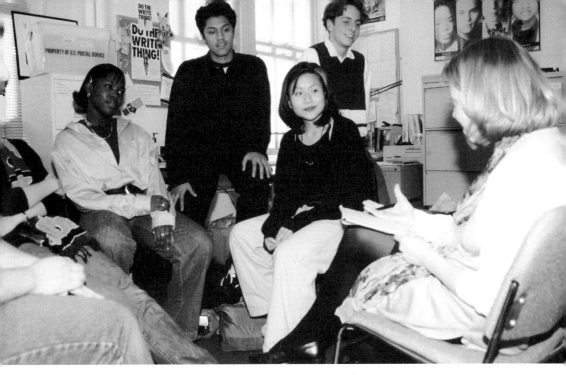

If you are troubled by your own alcohol use, or that of someone close to you, consider getting help.

have a car accident, or you get arrested, or injured, or hurt someone you care about, or your grades start to suffer. Being worried about your alcohol use is a sign that some aspect of it is troubling you. And if you are troubled by alcohol use, then you have a problem with alcohol.

How to Get Help

To get help, you need to find and reach out to someone you can trust. A family member or a friend might be a logical choice. But you also need to be aware of the possibility that it may have been problems with friends or family that led you to using alcohol in the first place. A teacher or school counselor, or some other adult you can trust, is also a good place to start. A doctor or therapist is someone else you could consult. Remember that alcoholism is a disease, and a disease often requires some kind of medical help before it gets better. Do not feel ashamed to ask for help.

There are numerous organizations devoted to helping those with chemical dependencies. Such organizations, called self-help groups, offer practical assistance and an atmosphere of emotional support. Being able to share your troubles and experiences with others who have undergone similar things is an important aspect of getting better. Perhaps the best-known such group of this kind is Alcoholics Anonymous (AA), which has chapters in thousands of communities across the country. Alateen is run by AA specifically for teens who have problems with alcohol and is one of AA's fastest growing programs. Your telephone book most likely contains the number of an advice or counseling line for alcohol or drug use. A trained counselor there can tell you how to get help.

You should also remember that it is possible to have a problem with alcohol use even if you do not drink. Having a family member, loved one, or friend who is an

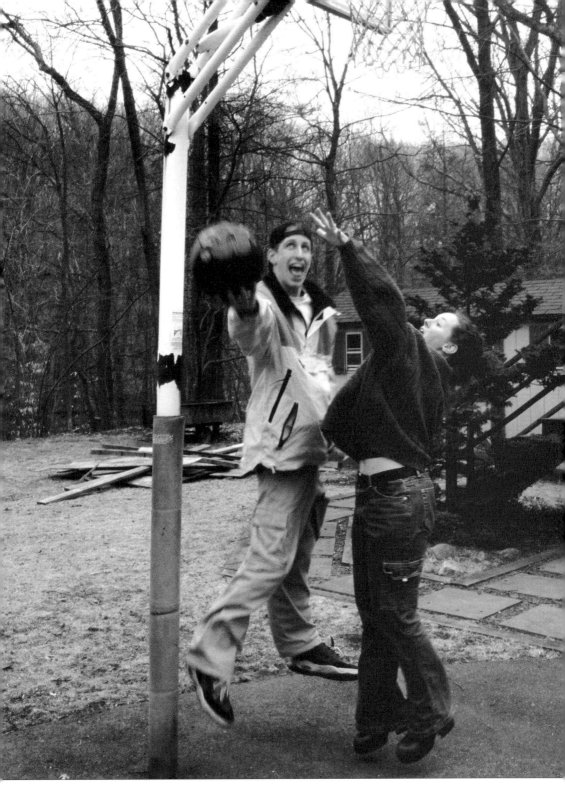

Finding positive activities that you enjoy is one of the most important steps to becoming emotionally healthy.

56 alcoholic can have a serious effect on you. Most self-help organizations also have programs for those who are negatively affected by the alcohol use of others. You cannot "save" someone who is an alcoholic. He or she has to do that for himself or herself. But you can help yourself.

You Are Not Alone

Finding a supportive environment, either with a medical professional or a self-help group, is the best way to take control of your alcohol use and also to begin to address the emotional issues that have contributed to your drinking. In reaching out, you will discover that you are not alone.

And despite what you may believe, you will also learn that not "everyone" drinks. Despite the alarming statistics, half of all teens do not use alcohol at all. (Nearly half of adults do not, either.) They find all kinds of interesting, fulfilling ways to spend their time. Indeed, one of the best ways to stay clear of alcohol is to find something that you love to do and to pursue it wholeheartedly. It could be an academic, athletic, or artistic interest—such as sports, music, dancing, or a school club. Doing something for others—as a volunteer through a church, shelter, hospital, or charitable organization—is enormously fulfilling.

There is simply no better way to make you feel good about yourself.

Most important, by reaching out and finding and pursuing your own interests, you usually have no choice but to make contact with others. And in time, you are bound to find that you have things in common with them—experiences, interests, backgrounds, thoughts, feelings, hopes, fears, and dreams. You will also discover that you do not need alcohol to share these things.

Glossary

alcoholism Chronic disease characterized by physical and psychological dependence on alcohol.

binge drinking The consumption of five or more alcoholic drinks in a row, over a short period of time.

COA Abbreviation for children of alcoholism.

date rape Sexual assault upon a woman by a man who is known to her.

dependency Addiction to a particular drug. Dependency has both a physical and a psychological component.

depressant A substance that slows down the way the body works.

domestic violence Violence that occurs in the home, usually between family members, often with women and children as the victims.

drug A substance that when ingested, changes a person's physical or emotional state through its effects on the body.

drunk A slang term for being intoxicated with alcohol or for an alcoholic.

fermentation Chemical process whereby yeast changes carbohydrates into ethyl alcohol and carbon dioxide.

gateway drug A drug whose use is believed to lead to the use of other drugs.

intoxicated Having enough alcohol in the bloodstream to interfere with judgment, behavior, or physical activity; the legal definition of intoxication is set by statute.

Prohibition Period of time in the United States, lasting from 1919 to 1933, in which the Eighteenth Amendment was in effect. The amendment prohibited the manufacture, sale, and use of alcoholic beverages.

psychoactive Affecting a person's perception of his or her physical or mental state.

tolerance Process of developing a reduced susceptibility to a drug's effects.

withdrawal Physical and psychological effects of stopping the use of a drug on which a person has become dependent.

Where to Go for Help

Al-Anon Family Groups
P.O. Box 862
Midtown Station
New York, NY 10018

Alcoholics Anonymous
P.O. Box 459
Grand Central Station
New York, NY 10163
(212) 870-3400
Web site: http://www.alcoholics-anonymous.org

Chemical People Project
WQED
4802 Fifth Avenue
Pittsburgh, PA 15213

The National Clearinghouse for Alcohol and Drug Information

P.O. Box 2345
Rockville, MD 20847-2345
(301) 468-2600
Web site: http://www/health.org

National Council on Alcoholism and Drug Dependence

12 West 21st Street
New York, NY 10010
(800) 622-2255
e-mail: national@NCADD.org

Youth Crisis Hotline

(800) 448-4663

In Canada

Alcohol and Drug Dependency Information and Counseling Services (ADDICS)

2471 1/2 Portage Avenue, #2
Winnipeg, Manitoba R3J ON6
(204) 942-4730

For Further Reading

Clayton, Lawrence. *Coping with a Drug-Abusing Parent.* New York: Rosen Publishing Group, 1995.

Fishman, Ross. *Alcohol and Alcoholism.* New York: Chelsea House, 1986.

Grosshandler, Janet. *Coping with Drinking and Driving.* New York: Rosen Publishing Group, 1997.

Hyde, Margaret O., and Bruce G. Hyde. *Know About Drugs.* New York: McGraw-Hill, 1979.

Madison, Arnold. *Drugs and You.* New York: Julian Messner, 1972.

Ryan, Elizabeth A. *Straight Talk About Drugs and Alcohol.* New York: Facts on File, 1989.

Shuker, Nancy. *Everything You Need to Know About an Alcoholic Parent.* New York: Rosen Publishing Group, 1998.

Taylor, Barbara. *Everything You Need to Know About Alcohol.* New York: Rosen Publishing Group, 1996.

Vogler, Roger E., and Wayne Bartz. *Teenagers and Alcohol: When Saying No Isn't Enough.* Philadelphia: The Charles Press, 1992.

Index

A

advertising, 6, 20
Alateen, 54
Alcoholics Anonymous (AA),
    54
alcoholism, 7–8, 20–21, 28,
    33–40, 47, 49, 54
anxiety disorders, 46

B

beer, 6, 14, 17, 19, 22, 48
binge drinking, 23–25

C

celebrations, 7, 43
children of alcoholics (COAs),
    20–21, 49
counselors, 20, 53–54, 56

D

decision making, 8–9, 20,
    30–31, 43, 47, 52
denial, 36
dependency, 32, 35–37, 45,
    49–50, 52, 54
    physical, 36–37
    psychological, 36–37
    stages of, 35–36
depression, 38–39, 41–43,
    46
"designated driver," 27
distilled liquors, 14, 48

E

effects of alcohol, 38
    on brain, 16–17, 18
    hangovers, 19
    on liver, 25, 29, 50
    loss of control, 17, 18, 36
    memory loss, 18, 35
    negative, 16–19, 20
    positive, 16
    on reflexes, 17, 18, 26
    vomiting, 18–19
ethyl alcohol, 14
experimenting, 33, 35, 38, 43

F

family/parents, 8, 9, 19, 27, 36,
    38, 39, 41–43, 44,
    45–46, 47, 49, 50, 53, 54
fermentation, 14
financial problems, 39–40, 45

G

guilt, 34

L

legality (of alcohol), 7, 15,
    26–27, 32
loneliness, 7, 42, 46

M

media images, 6, 9, 20
metabolism, 35, 50

64

P

parties, 8, 11–13, 18–19,
 22–23, 27, 30, 33–34
peer pressure, 46–47

R

relationships, 8, 36
religious ceremonies, 7
risk factors (for problems
 with alcohol), 48–51
risks/consequences (of alcohol
 use), 8–9, 13, 21,
 22–32, 43
 academic problems, 29,
 36, 39, 53
 accidents, 7, 23, 27, 28
 blackouts, 18, 35
 criminal behavior, 8, 31–32
 domestic violence, 7, 31
 drunk driving, 26–27, 28,
 32, 34, 53
 loss of consciousness, 18,
 22–23, 25
 overdosing, 23–25, 28
 sexual activity, 8, 30
 sexual assaults, 30, 31
 STDs (sexually transmitted
 diseases), 31

S

sale (of alcohol), 7
self-help groups, 54, 56
self-medication, 46
social drinking, 7, 16, 44

T

tolerance, 35

U

United States (use of alcohol
 in), 7, 15, 20–21,
 26–27, 28–29, 35

W

well-being, 16
wine, 6, 8, 14, 16, 48
withdrawal, 37

Y

yeast, 14

About the Author

Christine Bichler lives with her husband in Ypsilanti, Michigan, where she teaches college composition and literature. She holds a Master's degree in literature from Eastern Michigan University.

Photo Credits

Cover Photo by Michelle Edwards. P. 2 by Seth Dimmerman; p. 44 by Les Mills; pp. 39, 53 by Ira Fox; p. 50 by M. Moreno; p. 15 © T. Tracy/FPG International. All other photos by Michelle Edwards.